I0703458

50 yoga poses you can try at home

Franklin Fisher

Copyright © (2024) by Franklin Fisher

All rights reserved. No portion of this book may be reproduced, stored, in a retrieval system or transmitted in any format or by any means, electronical, mechanical, photocopying, recording, or otherwise, without the prior written permission of the author.

Published by Amazon KDP

Amazon.com, Inc.

P.O. Box 81226

Seattle, WA 98108-1226

United States.

Printed by Amazon KDP in the USA

Table of contents

Mountain Pose (Tadasana)

Mountain Pose (Tadasana) is a foundational yoga posture that serves as the starting position for many other poses. To perform Mountain Pose:

1. Stand tall with your feet hip-width apart, toes pointing forward, and arms relaxed by your sides.
2. Distribute your weight evenly on both feet and engage your leg muscles.
3. Lengthen your spine by lifting your chest and rolling your shoulders back and down.
4. Keep your chin parallel to the ground and gaze forward softly.
5. Press down through your feet, feeling rooted to the ground, while simultaneously reaching upward through the crown of your head.
6. Take slow, deep breaths, and hold the pose for 30 seconds to 1 minute, focusing on your alignment and breathing.

Downward-Facing Dog (Adho Mukha Svanasana)

Downward-Facing Dog, or Adho Mukha Svanasana in Sanskrit, is one of the most widely recognized yoga poses and is often practiced as part of a sun salutation sequence. Here's how to do it:

1. Begin on your hands and knees, with your wrists aligned under your shoulders and your knees under your hips.
2. Spread your fingers wide apart and press firmly into the mat with your palms, creating a strong foundation.
3. Tuck your toes under and exhale as you lift your hips toward the ceiling, straightening your arms and legs to form an inverted V shape.
4. Keep your hands shoulder-width apart and your feet hip-width apart. Your heels may or may not touch the mat, depending on your flexibility.
5. Lengthen your spine by reaching your tailbone toward the ceiling and pressing your chest toward your thighs.
6. Engage your quadriceps to lift your kneecaps and firm your thighs.

7. Relax your head and neck, allowing them to hang freely between your arms.
8. Press firmly into your palms and distribute your weight evenly between your hands and feet.
9. Hold the pose for 5-10 breaths, breathing deeply and evenly.
10. To release, exhale as you gently lower your knees back to the mat.

Downward-Facing Dog stretches the entire body, particularly the hamstrings, calves, shoulders, and spine. It also strengthens the arms, shoulders, and core muscles while calming the mind and relieving stress. Practice this pose regularly to improve flexibility, strength, and overall well-being.

Warrior I (Virabhadrasana I)

Warrior I, or Virabhadrasana I in Sanskrit, is a powerful standing pose that builds strength, stability, and focus. Here's how to practice it:

1. Begin in Mountain Pose (Tadasana) at the top of your mat, with your feet hip-width apart and arms by your sides.
2. Step your left foot back, keeping the toes pointed slightly outward at a 45-degree angle.
3. Bend your right knee, stacking it directly over your right ankle, so your shin is perpendicular to the floor. Your left leg should be straight and strong, with the heel pressing firmly into the mat.
4. Pivot your left foot slightly inward, about 45 degrees, to help square your hips toward the front of the mat.
5. Inhale as you raise your arms overhead, reaching upward with your fingertips, palms facing each other, or bringing your palms together.
6. Keep your shoulders relaxed and down away from your ears, and gaze forward or slightly upward.

7. Sink deeper into the bend of your right knee, ensuring it stays aligned with your ankle and doesn't extend past your toes.
8. Engage your core muscles to support your spine, and press firmly into the outer edge of your back foot.
9. Hold the pose for 30 seconds to 1 minute, breathing deeply and maintaining steady focus.
10. To release, exhale as you lower your arms and step your left foot forward to meet your right foot in Mountain Pose.

Warrior I strengthens the legs, arms, and core muscles while improving balance and concentration. It also opens the hips and chest, promoting a sense of confidence and empowerment. Practice this pose regularly to cultivate inner strength and resilience.

Warrior II (Virabhadrasana II)

Warrior II, or Virabhadrasana II in Sanskrit, is a dynamic standing pose that builds strength, stability, and focus while also promoting openness in the hips and chest. Here's how to practice it:

1. Begin in Mountain Pose (Tadasana) at the top of your mat, with your feet hip-width apart and arms by your sides.
2. Step your left foot back, keeping the toes pointed slightly outward at a 45-degree angle.
3. Extend your arms out to the sides at shoulder height, parallel to the floor, with your palms facing down.
4. Bend your right knee, stacking it directly over your right ankle, so your shin is perpendicular to the floor. Your left leg should be straight and strong, with the heel pressing firmly into the mat.
5. Pivot your left foot slightly inward, about 45 degrees, to help square your hips toward the side of the mat.

6. Gaze over your right fingertips, keeping your head aligned with your spine.
7. Relax your shoulders down away from your ears and engage your core muscles to support your spine.
8. Ensure your right knee stays aligned with your ankle and doesn't extend past your toes.
9. Press firmly into the outer edge of your back foot and keep both legs strong and active.
10. Hold the pose for 30 seconds to 1 minute, breathing deeply and maintaining steady focus.
11. To release, exhale as you straighten your right leg and lower your arms. Step your left foot forward to meet your right foot in Mountain Pose.

Warrior II strengthens the legs, arms, and core muscles while stretching the hips, groin, and chest. It also cultivates a sense of confidence, courage, and determination. Practice this pose regularly to build physical and mental resilience.

Warrior III (Virabhadrasana III)

Warrior III, or Virabhadrasana III in Sanskrit, is a challenging balancing pose that strengthens the legs, core, and back muscles while improving concentration and focus. Here's how to practice it:

1. Begin in Mountain Pose (Tadasana) at the top of your mat, with your feet hip-width apart and arms by your sides.
2. Shift your weight onto your right foot and ground down through the entire foot, spreading your toes for stability.
3. On an inhale, lift your left leg off the mat behind you, keeping it straight and parallel to the floor. Point your toes toward the back of the mat.
4. Simultaneously, begin to hinge forward at your hips, lowering your torso until it is parallel to the floor. Keep your spine straight and your chest lifted.
5. Extend your arms out in front of you, parallel to the floor, with your palms facing each other. Engage your core muscles to maintain balance.

6. Keep your standing leg strong and straight, with a slight micro-bend in the knee to avoid locking it.

7. Ensure your hips are squared toward the mat, with your left hip pointing down.

8. Lengthen through the crown of your head and reach back through your left heel to create a straight line from your head to your left foot.

9. Find a focal point (drishti) on the floor a few feet in front of you to help maintain your balance and focus.

10. Hold the pose for 5-10 breaths, breathing deeply and evenly.

11. To release, exhale as you slowly lower your left leg to the mat and come back to Mountain Pose.

12. Repeat on the other side, shifting your weight onto your left foot and lifting your right leg.

Warrior III improves balance, coordination, and proprioception while strengthening the legs, core, and back muscles. It also encourages mental focus and concentration. Practice this pose regularly to develop stability and poise both on and off the mat.

Tree Pose (Vrksasana)

Tree Pose, or Vrksasana in Sanskrit, is a balancing pose that cultivates stability, focus, and calmness. Here's how to practice it:

1. Begin in Mountain Pose (Tadasana) at the top of your mat, with your feet hip-width apart and arms by your sides.
2. Shift your weight onto your right foot and ground down through the entire foot, spreading your toes for stability.
3. On an inhale, bend your left knee and reach down to grab your left ankle with your left hand.
4. Place the sole of your left foot on the inner thigh or calf of your right leg, avoiding placing it directly on the knee joint.
5. Press the sole of your left foot firmly into the inner thigh or calf, and the inner thigh or calf into the sole of your foot, creating a strong connection.
6. Engage your core muscles to maintain stability and lengthen through your spine, lifting your chest and rolling your shoulders back and down.
7. Bring your palms together in front of your heart in a prayer position, or

extend your arms overhead with your palms facing each other.

8. Find a focal point (drishti) on the floor or wall in front of you to help maintain your balance and focus.
9. Keep your gaze steady and soft, and your breath smooth and steady.
10. Hold the pose for 30 seconds to 1 minute, breathing deeply and evenly.
11. To release, exhale as you gently lower your left foot to the mat and return to Mountain Pose.
12. Repeat on the other side, shifting your weight onto your left foot and bringing your right foot to rest on the inner thigh or calf of your left leg.

Tree Pose strengthens the muscles of the standing leg, while also improving balance, posture, and concentration. It opens the hips and stretches the inner thighs and groin, promoting a sense of groundedness and connection to the earth. Practice this pose regularly to cultivate balance and harmony in both body and mind.

Chair Pose (Utkatasana)

Chair Pose, or Utkatasana in Sanskrit, is a powerful standing pose that strengthens the legs, glutes, and core muscles while promoting stability and focus. Here's how to practice it:

1. Begin in Mountain Pose (Tadasana) at the top of your mat, with your feet hip-width apart and arms by your sides.
2. On an inhale, raise your arms overhead, palms facing each other or coming together in a prayer position.
3. Exhale as you bend your knees and lower your hips back and down as if you were sitting back into a chair. Keep your knees aligned with your ankles, and shift your weight into your heels.
4. Engage your core muscles to support your lower back and keep your spine straight. Lengthen through your tailbone and lift your chest slightly.
5. Keep your arms reaching upward, with your biceps alongside your ears and your shoulders relaxed away from your ears.

6. Gaze forward or slightly upward, finding a focal point to help maintain your balance and focus.
7. Press firmly into your feet, especially your heels, to activate the muscles of your legs and glutes.
8. Hold the pose for 30 seconds to 1 minute, breathing deeply and evenly.
9. To release, exhale as you straighten your legs and lower your arms back down to your sides, returning to Mountain Pose.

Chair Pose strengthens the quadriceps, hamstrings, calves, and glutes, while also improving ankle stability and mobility. It engages the core muscles, promoting better posture and spinal alignment. Practice this pose regularly to build strength, endurance, and mental resilience.

Child's Pose (Balasana)

Child's Pose, or Balasana in Sanskrit, is a gentle resting pose that stretches the back, hips, thighs, and ankles while promoting relaxation and grounding. Here's how to practice it:

1. Begin by kneeling on the mat with your knees hip-width apart and your big toes touching behind you.
2. Sit back on your heels, keeping your spine long and your shoulders relaxed.
3. On an exhale, slowly lower your torso forward, bringing your forehead to rest on the mat in front of your knees.
4. Extend your arms out in front of you, palms facing down, or bring them alongside your body with your palms facing up, whichever is more comfortable.
5. Relax your entire body into the pose, allowing your hips to sink toward your heels and your chest to rest on or between your thighs.
6. Close your eyes if comfortable, and let your forehead rest on the mat, releasing any tension in your neck and shoulders.

7. Take slow, deep breaths, feeling the gentle expansion of your back with each inhale and the release of tension with each exhale.

8. Stay in Child's Pose for as long as feels comfortable, anywhere from 1 to 5 minutes or longer.

9. To release, gently walk your hands back toward your body, lifting your torso upright and sitting back on your heels.

Child's Pose is a soothing posture that calms the mind and relieves stress and fatigue. It gently stretches the spine, hips, thighs, and ankles, providing a gentle release for tension accumulated throughout the day. Use this pose as a resting position during your yoga practice or anytime you need a moment of relaxation and rejuvenation.

Cobra Pose (Bhujangasana)

Cobra Pose, or Bhujangasana in Sanskrit, is a rejuvenating backbend that strengthens the spine, opens the chest and shoulders, and improves posture. Here's how to practice it:

1. Begin by lying flat on your stomach, with your legs extended behind you and the tops of your feet resting on the mat.
2. Place your palms on the mat next to your ribcage, fingertips in line with your chest and elbows pointing back and close to your body.
3. Press down through the tops of your feet and pubic bone, engaging your leg muscles and pelvic floor.
4. On an inhale, gently press into your hands and lift your chest off the mat, using the strength of your back muscles.
5. Keep your elbows bent and close to your sides, with your shoulders relaxed away from your ears.
6. Lengthen through your spine, reaching your tailbone toward your heels and lifting your sternum toward the ceiling.

7. Keep your gaze forward or slightly upward, without compressing the back of your neck.
8. Press firmly into your hands to lift your chest higher, while also drawing your shoulder blades down and back to open your chest.
9. Hold the pose for 15-30 seconds, breathing deeply and evenly.
10. To release, exhale as you slowly lower your chest back down to the mat, resting your forehead on the ground.

Cobra Pose strengthens the muscles of the back, arms, and core, while also improving spinal flexibility and relieving tension in the lower back. It stimulates the organs in the abdomen and can be therapeutic for mild back pain. Practice this pose mindfully, focusing on maintaining length and integrity in the spine while avoiding excessive compression in the lower back.

Cat-Cow Stretch (Marjaryasana-Bitilasana)

The Cat-Cow Stretch, also known as Marjaryasana-Bitilasana in Sanskrit, is a gentle and flowing movement that stretches and mobilizes the spine while also promoting flexibility and coordination. Here's how to practice it:

1. Begin on your hands and knees in a tabletop position, with your wrists directly under your shoulders and your knees directly under your hips.
2. Keep your spine neutral and your neck in line with your spine, with your gaze directed toward the mat.
3. On an inhale, arch your back and tilt your pelvis down, lifting your chest and tailbone toward the ceiling. This is the Cow Pose (Bitilasana).
4. At the same time, lift your head and chest slightly, allowing your belly to sink toward the floor, creating a gentle backbend.
5. Hold the Cow Pose for a few breaths, feeling a stretch through the front of your torso and opening through your chest and shoulders.

6. On an exhale, round your spine upward, tucking your chin toward your chest and drawing your belly button toward your spine. This is the Cat Pose (Marjaryasana).
7. Press firmly into your hands and knees as you round your back, creating space between your shoulder blades and drawing your tailbone toward your knees.
8. Hold the Cat Pose for a few breaths, feeling a stretch through your upper back and releasing tension in your spine.
9. Continue to flow between Cat and Cow Poses, moving with your breath. Inhale to arch into Cow Pose, and exhale to round into Cat Pose.
10. Repeat this flowing movement for 5-10 rounds, allowing your breath to guide the rhythm of the movement.
11. After your final round, return to a neutral tabletop position.

The Cat-Cow Stretch gently warms up the spine, increases flexibility, and releases tension in the back, neck, and shoulders. It also massages and stimulates the organs in the abdomen, promoting digestion and relaxation. Practice this stretch regularly, especially at the beginning of your yoga practice or as a standalone sequence to help alleviate stiffness and improve spinal mobility.

Bridge Pose (Setu Bandhasana)

Bridge Pose, or Setu Bandhasana in Sanskrit, is a rejuvenating backbend that strengthens the back, glutes, and legs while opening the chest and shoulders. Here's how to practice it:

1. Begin by lying flat on your back, with your knees bent and feet hip-width apart on the mat. Your arms should be resting alongside your body with palms facing down.
2. Press your feet into the mat, engaging your glutes and hamstrings.
3. On an inhale, lift your hips toward the ceiling by pressing into your feet and arms.
4. Keep your knees directly over your ankles, and your thighs parallel to each other.
5. Roll your shoulders back and down, and press your upper arms into the mat to lift your chest toward your chin.
6. Interlace your fingers underneath your back, and press your arms into the mat to lift your chest even higher.
7. Keep your chin slightly tucked to lengthen the back of your neck, and

gaze straight ahead or toward your knees.

8. Hold the pose for 30 seconds to 1 minute, breathing deeply and evenly.
9. To release, unclasp your hands and slowly lower your spine back down to the mat, one vertebra at a time.

Bridge Pose strengthens the muscles of the back, glutes, and legs, while also stretching the chest, neck, and spine. It stimulates the abdominal organs, improves digestion, and can help alleviate mild back pain. Practice this pose regularly to build strength and flexibility in the back body, and to promote a sense of openness and vitality.

Plank Pose (Phalakasana)

Plank Pose, or Phalakasana in Sanskrit, is a foundational yoga pose that builds strength in the core, arms, shoulders, and wrists. Here's how to practice it:

1. Begin on your hands and knees in a tabletop position, with your wrists directly under your shoulders and your knees directly under your hips.
2. Spread your fingers wide apart and press firmly into the mat with your palms, creating a strong foundation for the pose.
3. Step your feet back one at a time, straightening your legs and aligning your heels with your hips. Your body should form a straight line from your head to your heels.
4. Engage your core muscles to support your spine and prevent your lower back from sagging.
5. Keep your shoulders stacked directly over your wrists, and your neck in line with your spine, with your gaze directed slightly forward.
6. Press firmly into the mat with your hands and lift through your forearms,

creating space between your shoulder blades.

7. Lengthen through the crown of your head and reach back through your heels, maintaining a strong and stable plank position.
8. Hold the pose for 30 seconds to 1 minute, breathing deeply and evenly.
9. To release, gently lower your knees to the mat and rest in Child's Pose or come back to a tabletop position.

Plank Pose strengthens the muscles of the core, including the abdominals, obliques, and lower back, while also toning the arms, shoulders, and chest. It improves posture, stability, and overall body awareness, making it an essential pose in any yoga or fitness routine. Practice plank regularly to build strength and endurance, and to cultivate a strong and stable foundation for your yoga practice.

Boat Pose (Navasana)

Boat Pose, or Navasana in Sanskrit, is a challenging yoga pose that strengthens the core muscles, including the abdominals and hip flexors, while also improving balance and focus. Here's how to practice it:

1. Begin by sitting on the mat with your knees bent and your feet flat on the floor, hip-width apart.
2. Place your hands behind your thighs, near your knees, with your fingers pointing toward your feet.
3. Lean back slightly and lift your feet off the floor, bringing your shins parallel to the mat.
4. Keep your knees bent initially to find your balance, and then straighten your legs as you feel stable.
5. Engage your core muscles to lift your chest and lengthen your spine, avoiding rounding in the upper back.
6. Extend your arms forward, parallel to the floor, with your palms facing each other.
7. Keep your shoulders relaxed away from your ears, and your chest lifted.

8. Find a focal point (drishti) in front of you to help maintain your balance and focus.
9. Hold the pose for 10-30 seconds, breathing deeply and evenly.
10. To release, exhale as you gently lower your feet back to the mat, returning to a seated position.

Boat Pose strengthens the muscles of the abdomen, hip flexors, and lower back, while also improving digestion and stimulating the organs in the abdomen. It requires concentration and mindfulness to maintain balance, making it a great pose for improving mental focus and stability. Practice Boat Pose regularly to build core strength and cultivate a sense of inner strength and stability.

Corpse Pose (Savasana)

Corpse Pose, or Savasana in Sanskrit, is a deeply relaxing and rejuvenating yoga pose that allows the body and mind to fully relax and integrate the benefits of your yoga practice. Here's how to practice it:

1. Lie down on your back on the mat, with your legs extended and your arms resting alongside your body, palms facing up.
2. Allow your feet to fall open naturally, with your toes pointing outward.
3. Keep your legs and arms slightly separated from your body, allowing for a feeling of spaciousness and relaxation.
4. Close your eyes gently, allowing your eyelids to feel heavy.
5. Take a few deep breaths, inhaling deeply through your nose and exhaling fully through your mouth, releasing any tension or stress with each exhale.
6. Relax your facial muscles, jaw, and tongue, allowing them to soften and release any remaining tension.
7. Bring your awareness to each part of your body, starting from your toes

and moving upward toward your head.

8. Scan your body for any areas of tension or discomfort, and consciously release and let go of any tension you find.
9. Allow your body to become heavy and sink into the mat, feeling supported and grounded.
10. Let go of any thoughts or worries, and simply focus on the sensation of your breath moving in and out of your body.
11. Remain in Corpse Pose for 5-10 minutes or longer, allowing yourself to fully surrender to relaxation and stillness.
12. When you're ready to come out of the pose, gently wiggle your fingers and toes, and slowly deepen your breath.
13. Roll onto your right side, using your right arm as a pillow for your head, and take a few moments to rest and integrate the benefits of your practice.
14. When you feel ready, slowly press yourself up to a seated position, keeping your eyes closed if possible.

Corpse Pose allows the body and mind to rest deeply, promoting relaxation, stress relief, and a sense of inner peace. It also allows for the integration of the physical, mental, and emotional benefits of your yoga practice, making it an essential and rejuvenating pose to conclude your practice with. Practice Corpse Pose regularly to cultivate a deeper sense of relaxation and well-being in your life.

Seated Forward Bend (Paschimottanasana)

Seated Forward Bend, or Paschimottanasana in Sanskrit, is a calming yoga pose that stretches the entire back body, including the spine, hamstrings, and calves, while also calming the mind and relieving stress. Here's how to practice it:

1. Begin by sitting on the mat with your legs extended straight in front of you and your feet flexed, toes pointing toward the ceiling.
2. Sit up tall with your spine lengthened, and engage your core muscles to support your lower back.
3. On an inhale, reach your arms overhead, lengthening through your fingertips toward the ceiling.
4. Exhale as you hinge forward at your hips, leading with your chest, and reach your hands toward your feet.
5. Keep your spine long as you fold forward, avoiding rounding in your back. Imagine leading with your heart rather than your head.
6. Place your hands wherever they comfortably reach – on your shins,

ankles, or feet – avoiding pulling or forcing the stretch.

7. Relax your neck and shoulders, allowing them to soften and release any tension.

8. Keep your feet flexed and your legs engaged, with your kneecaps lifting toward the ceiling to protect your hamstrings.

9. If you're able to go deeper into the stretch, you can walk your hands further down your legs or reach for the outsides of your feet.

10. Hold the pose for 30 seconds to 1 minute, breathing deeply and evenly.

11. To release, inhale as you slowly lift your torso back up to a seated position, lengthening through your spine.

Seated Forward Bend provides a deep stretch to the entire back body, including the spine, hamstrings, and calves, while also calming the nervous system and promoting relaxation. It can help relieve tension in the back and improve posture, flexibility, and digestion. Practice this pose regularly, focusing on deep, mindful breathing and maintaining a sense of ease and relaxation in the posture.

Garland Pose (Malasana)

Garland Pose, or Malasana in Sanskrit, is a grounding yoga pose that stretches the ankles, hips, groin, and lower back while also strengthening the legs and opening the chest. Here's how to practice it:

1. Begin by standing at the top of your mat with your feet slightly wider than hip-width apart.
2. Turn your toes out slightly, so they point toward the corners of your mat.
3. Bend your knees deeply and lower your hips toward the mat, coming into a squat position.
4. Bring your palms together at your heart center in a prayer position, pressing your elbows against your inner knees to gently open your hips.
5. Keep your spine long and your chest lifted, avoiding rounding in your back.
6. Press your hands together firmly, engaging your arm muscles, and use your elbows to gently push your knees back, creating space in your hips.
7. If possible, bring your heels to the mat, keeping them in line with your

toes. If your heels don't reach the mat, you can place a folded blanket or yoga block underneath them for support.

8. Press firmly into your feet and lift through your chest, finding length in your spine.
9. Hold the pose for 30 seconds to 1 minute, breathing deeply and evenly.
10. To release, exhale as you bring your hands to the mat in front of you, straighten your legs, and come back to a standing position.

Garland Pose stretches the ankles, hips, groin, and lower back, while also strengthening the legs and opening the chest. It stimulates the digestive organs and can help improve digestion and elimination. Practice this pose regularly to increase flexibility in the hips and lower back, and to cultivate a sense of grounding and stability in your yoga practice.

Triangle Pose (Trikonasana)

Triangle Pose, or Trikonasana in Sanskrit, is a classic yoga pose that stretches and strengthens the legs, hips, spine, and shoulders while also improving balance and concentration. Here's how to practice it:

1. Begin by standing at the top of your mat with your feet about 3-4 feet apart, parallel to each other.
2. Turn your right foot out 90 degrees, so your right toes point to the top of your mat. Keep your left foot turned in slightly, about 45 degrees.
3. Extend your arms out to the sides at shoulder height, palms facing down, with your shoulders relaxed away from your ears.
4. On an inhale, reach your right arm forward as you hinge at your right hip and lower your right hand toward your right shin, ankle, or the floor, whichever is accessible to you. You can also place a block on the outside of your right foot for support.
5. Keep your left arm reaching up toward the ceiling, with your chest and hips open toward the side of your mat.

6. Align your shoulders so they stack directly over each other, and gaze up toward your left fingertips.
7. Keep your legs engaged and strong, with your thighs lifting upward and your kneecaps lifting toward your hips.
8. Press down firmly through the outer edge of your left foot and the inner edge of your right foot to maintain stability.
9. Lengthen through your spine, reaching your tailbone toward your left heel and the crown of your head toward the front of your mat.
10. Hold the pose for 30 seconds to 1 minute, breathing deeply and evenly.
11. To release, inhale as you press into your feet and reach your left arm up to return to a standing position. Then, repeat on the other side.

Triangle Pose stretches the hamstrings, groins, hips, spine, and shoulders, while also strengthening the legs, core, and back muscles. It stimulates the abdominal organs and can help improve digestion and relieve stress.

Practice this pose regularly to increase flexibility, strength, and balance, while also cultivating a sense of openness and stability in your yoga practice.

Extended Side Angle Pose (Utthita Parsvakonasana)

Extended Side Angle Pose, or Utthita Parsvakonasana in Sanskrit, is a dynamic yoga pose that stretches and strengthens the legs, hips, spine, and shoulders while also improving balance and concentration. Here's how to practice it:

1. Begin by standing at the top of your mat in Mountain Pose (Tadasana), with your feet together and your arms by your sides.
2. Step your feet wide apart, about 3-4 feet, turning your right foot out 90 degrees and your left foot in slightly, about 45 degrees.
3. On an inhale, reach your arms out to the sides at shoulder height, palms facing down, and gaze over your right fingertips.
4. On an exhale, bend your right knee, stacking it directly over your right ankle, so your thigh is parallel to the floor. Keep your left leg straight and strong.
5. Bring your right hand to the inside of your right foot, either placing it on the floor, a block, or your shin, depending

on your flexibility. Your right forearm can also rest on your thigh for support.

6. Reach your left arm up toward the ceiling, with your biceps alongside your left ear and your palm facing down. Your left shoulder should be stacked directly over your right shoulder.

7. Keep your chest and hips open toward the side of your mat, with your spine lengthened and your tailbone reaching toward your left heel.

8. Engage your core muscles to support your spine, and keep your legs strong and engaged.

9. Press down firmly through the outer edge of your left foot and the inner edge of your right foot to maintain stability.

10. Hold the pose for 30 seconds to 1 minute, breathing deeply and evenly.

11. To release, inhale as you press into your feet and reach your left arm up to return to a standing position. Then, repeat on the other side.

Extended Side Angle Pose stretches the groin, hamstrings, hips, spine, and shoulders, while also strengthening the legs, core, and back muscles. It stimulates the abdominal organs and can help improve digestion and relieve stress. Practice this pose regularly to increase flexibility, strength, and balance, while also cultivating a sense of openness and stability in your yoga practice.

Extended Puppy Pose (Uttana Shishosana)

Extended Puppy Pose, or Uttana Shishosana in Sanskrit, is a gentle and soothing yoga pose that stretches the spine, shoulders, and arms while also relieving tension in the neck and upper back. Here's how to practice it:

1. Begin on your hands and knees in a tabletop position, with your wrists directly under your shoulders and your knees directly under your hips.
2. Walk your hands forward, keeping your arms shoulder-width apart, and lower your chest and forehead toward the mat.
3. Keep your hips stacked over your knees and your arms extended, with your palms pressing firmly into the mat.
4. Relax your forehead on the mat, allowing your neck to lengthen and your shoulders to soften.
5. Keep your hips lifted slightly to maintain a gentle stretch in the spine.
6. If your forehead doesn't reach the mat, you can place a folded blanket or yoga block underneath it for support.

7. Press down through your palms and fingertips to lengthen your arms and create space in your shoulders.
8. Stay in the pose for 1-3 minutes, breathing deeply and evenly.
9. To release, walk your hands back toward your body, coming back to a tabletop position.

Extended Puppy Pose stretches the spine, shoulders, and arms, while also opening the chest and heart center. It can help relieve tension and tightness in the upper back and neck, making it especially beneficial for those who spend long hours sitting or working at a desk. Practice this pose regularly to promote relaxation and relieve stress in the body and mind.

Reclining Bound Angle Pose (Supta Baddha Konasana)

Reclining Bound Angle Pose, or Supta Baddha Konasana in Sanskrit, is a restorative yoga pose that opens the hips, groin, and chest while promoting relaxation and stress relief. Here's how to practice it:

1. Begin by sitting on the mat with your knees bent and your feet flat on the floor, hip-width apart.
2. Bring the soles of your feet together and allow your knees to fall open to the sides, creating a diamond shape with your legs.
3. Slide your feet away from your body until you feel a gentle stretch in your inner thighs and groin. You can adjust the distance between your feet to find a comfortable position.
4. Lower your torso back onto the mat, supporting yourself with your hands as you recline.
5. Allow your arms to rest alongside your body, palms facing up, with your shoulders relaxed and your chest open.

6. Close your eyes and take slow, deep breaths, allowing your body to relax and soften with each exhale.
7. If you have props available, you can place a folded blanket or bolster under your knees for support, or a bolster or rolled-up blanket behind your back for added comfort.
8. Stay in the pose for 1-5 minutes, or longer if desired, breathing deeply and allowing yourself to surrender fully to relaxation.
9. To release, gently press your palms into the mat and use your hands to help bring your knees together.
10. Hug your knees into your chest and gently rock from side to side to release any tension in your lower back.
11. Roll onto your right side and rest there for a few breaths before slowly coming back up to a seated position.

Reclining Bound Angle Pose gently opens the hips and groin, stretches the inner thighs, and relieves tension in the lower back and pelvis. It can also help alleviate menstrual discomfort and improve circulation in the pelvic region. Practice this pose regularly, especially at the end of your yoga practice or before bedtime, to promote deep relaxation and restore balance to the body and mind.

Pigeon Pose (Eka Pada Rajakapotasana)

Pigeon Pose, or Eka Pada Rajakapotasana in Sanskrit, is a deep hip-opening yoga pose that stretches the hips, thighs, and groin while also releasing tension in the lower back and pelvis. Here's how to practice it:

1. Begin in a tabletop position on the mat, with your wrists directly under your shoulders and your knees directly under your hips.
2. On an exhale, slide your right knee forward toward your right wrist, bringing it to the outer edge of your mat. Your right shin should be angled diagonally across your mat, with your right foot flexed.
3. Slide your left leg back behind you, straightening it as much as possible, and lower your hips toward the mat. Keep your left hip squared toward the front of your mat.
4. Ensure your right knee is aligned with your right wrist, and your right foot is flexed to protect your knee.
5. If you're comfortable and want to deepen the stretch, you can walk your hands forward and lower your upper

body toward the mat, resting on your forearms or forehead.

6. Keep your spine long and your chest lifted, avoiding rounding in your back.
7. Hold the pose for 1-3 minutes, breathing deeply and evenly.
8. To release, press into your palms and slowly walk your hands back toward your body, lifting your chest and coming back to a tabletop position.
9. Repeat the pose on the other side, bringing your left knee forward and your right leg back.

Pigeon Pose stretches the hips, thighs, and groin, while also releasing tension in the lower back and pelvis. It can help improve hip flexibility and alleviate discomfort from prolonged sitting or tight hips. Practice this pose regularly, being mindful of any discomfort or sensation of pinching in the knee, and use props such as a blanket or block for support if needed.

Camel Pose (Ustrasana)

Camel Pose, or Ustrasana in Sanskrit, is an energizing backbend that stretches the front of the body, including the chest, abdomen, and hip flexors, while also strengthening the back muscles and improving spinal flexibility. Here's how to practice it:

1. Begin by kneeling on the mat with your knees hip-width apart and your thighs perpendicular to the floor. Keep your shins and feet relaxed on the mat, with the tops of your feet pressing into the ground.
2. Place your hands on your lower back, with your fingers pointing downward and your palms resting on your sacrum. Your fingertips should be pointing toward your tailbone.
3. On an inhale, lengthen through your spine and lift your chest toward the ceiling, gently arching your back.
4. Press your hips forward slightly, engaging your glutes and thighs to support your lower back.
5. Keep your shoulders relaxed away from your ears and your chin parallel to the floor.

6. If you feel comfortable, you can begin to reach your hands one at a time toward your heels, bringing your palms to rest on your heels or the soles of your feet.
7. Keep your thighs and hips pressing forward as you continue to lift your chest toward the ceiling, opening through the front of your body.
8. Hold the pose for 15-30 seconds, breathing deeply and evenly.
9. To release, bring your hands back to your lower back, slowly tuck your chin toward your chest, and lower your torso back down to a kneeling position.

Camel Pose stretches the front of the body, including the chest, abdomen, and hip flexors, while also strengthening the back muscles and improving spinal flexibility. It can help improve posture, relieve tension in the neck and shoulders, and stimulate the organs in the abdomen. Practice this pose mindfully, listening to your body and only going as deep into the pose as feels comfortable for you.

Sphinx Pose (Salamba Bhujangasana)

Sphinx Pose, or Salamba Bhujangasana in Sanskrit, is a gentle backbend that stretches the spine, chest, and shoulders while also strengthening the muscles of the back. Here's how to practice it:

1. Begin by lying flat on your stomach on the mat, with your legs extended behind you and the tops of your feet resting on the floor.
2. Place your forearms on the mat parallel to each other, with your elbows directly under your shoulders and your palms pressing into the mat.
3. Keep your elbows close to your body and your forearms parallel to each other, with your fingertips pointing forward.
4. On an inhale, press into your forearms and lift your chest and head off the mat, drawing your shoulders back and down.
5. Keep your gaze forward and slightly upward, with your neck in line with your spine.
6. Engage your core muscles to support your lower back, and press down

through the tops of your feet to lift your legs slightly off the mat.

7. Keep your hips grounded and your buttocks relaxed as you continue to lift through your chest.
8. Hold the pose for 15-30 seconds, breathing deeply and evenly.
9. To release, exhale as you gently lower your chest and head back down to the mat, resting your forehead on the ground.

Sphinx Pose stretches the spine, chest, and shoulders, while also strengthening the muscles of the back and improving posture. It can help relieve tension in the lower back and promote flexibility and mobility in the spine. Practice this pose regularly, focusing on lengthening through the spine and opening through the chest, to cultivate a sense of ease and spaciousness in the body and mind.

Upward-Facing Dog (Urdhva Mukha Svanasana)

Upward-Facing Dog, or Urdhva Mukha Svanasana in Sanskrit, is an invigorating backbend that strengthens the arms, shoulders, and back while also stretching the chest and abdomen. Here's how to practice it:

1. Begin by lying flat on your stomach on the mat, with your legs extended behind you and the tops of your feet pressing into the floor.
2. Place your palms on the mat next to your ribcage, with your fingertips in line with your chest and your elbows pointing upward and close to your body.
3. On an inhale, press into your palms and lift your chest and head off the mat, straightening your arms and lifting your torso upward.
4. Keep your shoulders stacked directly over your wrists, and your arms straight and strong.
5. Press down through the tops of your feet and lift your thighs and knees off the mat, engaging your leg muscles.

6. Keep your elbows bent slightly, and draw your shoulder blades down and back to open your chest.
7. Lift through your sternum and gaze forward, without compressing the back of your neck.
8. Keep your buttocks firm but not clenched, and your tailbone lengthening toward your heels.
9. Hold the pose for 15-30 seconds, breathing deeply and evenly.
10. To release, exhale as you slowly lower your chest and head back down to the mat, resting your forehead on the ground.

Upward-Facing Dog strengthens the arms, shoulders, and back muscles, while also stretching the chest and abdomen. It improves posture, opens the heart center, and stimulates the organs in the abdomen. Practice this pose mindfully, focusing on lengthening through the spine and opening through the chest, to cultivate strength, flexibility, and vitality in the body and mind.

Fish Pose (Matsyasana)

Fish Pose, or Matsyasana in Sanskrit, is a gentle backbend that stretches the chest, throat, and abdomen while also stimulating the thyroid gland and opening the heart center. Here's how to practice it:

1. Begin by lying flat on your back on the mat, with your legs extended and your arms resting alongside your body, palms facing down.
2. Slide your hands underneath your hips, palms facing down, with your elbows tucked in close to your body.
3. On an inhale, press into your forearms and lift your chest upward, arching your back and bringing the crown of your head toward the mat.
4. Keep your legs active and engaged, pressing through your heels and pointing your toes toward the ceiling.
5. Relax your buttocks and allow your weight to rest on your forearms and elbows, rather than on the crown of your head.
6. Tilt your head back slightly and allow your throat to open, breathing deeply and evenly.

7. If you're comfortable, you can lift your chest even higher, coming up onto the crown of your head and resting the back of your head on the mat.
8. Keep your shoulders relaxed away from your ears and your chest open.
9. Hold the pose for 15-30 seconds, breathing deeply and evenly.
10. To release, exhale as you slowly lower your chest and head back down to the mat, releasing your arms from underneath you and resting in Corpse Pose (Savasana) for a few breaths.

Fish Pose stretches the chest, throat, and abdomen, while also stimulating the thyroid gland and opening the heart center. It can help improve posture, relieve tension in the neck and shoulders, and alleviate fatigue. Practice this pose regularly, focusing on deep, mindful breathing and opening through the chest, to cultivate a sense of openness and vitality in the body and mind.

Half Moon Pose (Ardha Chandrasana)

Half Moon Pose, or Ardha Chandrasana in Sanskrit, is a dynamic balancing pose that strengthens the legs, core, and ankles while also improving coordination and focus. Here's how to practice it:

1. Begin in a standing position at the top of your mat, with your feet together and your arms by your sides in Mountain Pose (Tadasana).
2. Shift your weight into your left foot and lift your right foot off the mat, coming into a standing balance on your left foot.
3. Bend your left knee slightly and hinge forward at your hips, bringing your torso parallel to the floor.
4. Place your left hand on the mat or on a block directly underneath your left shoulder, about a foot in front of your left foot.
5. Keep your left fingertips in line with your left toes, and your left wrist directly under your left shoulder.
6. Extend your right leg straight out behind you, parallel to the floor, with

your right foot flexed and your toes pointing toward the floor.

7. Stack your right hip over your left hip and keep your right shoulder stacked over your left shoulder, creating a straight line from your fingertips to your right heel.
8. Engage your core muscles to support your spine and pelvis, and keep your gaze directed toward the floor or slightly forward.
9. If you feel stable, you can lift your right arm toward the ceiling, reaching it up alongside your ear, with your palm facing forward.
10. Hold the pose for 15-30 seconds, breathing deeply and evenly.
11. To release, exhale as you slowly lower your right hand and right foot back to the mat, coming back to a standing position at the top of your mat.
12. Repeat the pose on the other side, balancing on your right foot and extending your left leg behind you.

Half Moon Pose strengthens the legs, core, and ankles, while also improving balance, coordination, and focus. It stretches the groins, hamstrings, and spine, and can help improve digestion and relieve stress. Practice this pose regularly, focusing on stability and alignment, to cultivate strength, balance, and grace in your yoga practice.

Eagle Pose (Garudasana)

Eagle Pose, or Garudasana in Sanskrit, is a balancing pose that stretches the shoulders, upper back, thighs, and calves while also improving concentration and focus. Here's how to practice it:

1. Begin standing tall at the top of your mat in Mountain Pose (Tadasana), with your arms by your sides and your feet hip-width apart.
2. Shift your weight onto your left foot and bend your knees slightly.
3. Lift your right leg and cross it over your left thigh, wrapping your right foot around your left calf if possible. You can also hook your right toes behind your left ankle for support if needed.
4. Balance on your left foot and sink down slightly into a half-squat position.
5. Extend your arms straight out in front of you at shoulder height, parallel to the floor.
6. Cross your right arm under your left arm, bending both elbows, and bring your palms together in front of your

face. Your elbows should be stacked over each other.

7. Keep your shoulders relaxed away from your ears and your gaze focused on a point in front of you to help maintain your balance.
8. Engage your core muscles to support your spine and pelvis, and keep your chest lifted.
9. If you're comfortable, you can sink down deeper into the squat position, lowering your hips toward the floor.
10. Hold the pose for 15-30 seconds, breathing deeply and evenly.
11. To release, gently unwind your arms and legs and come back to a standing position.
12. Repeat the pose on the other side, balancing on your right foot and crossing your left leg over your right thigh.

Eagle Pose stretches the shoulders, upper back, thighs, and calves, while also improving balance, concentration, and focus. It can help relieve tension in the shoulders and upper back and improve mobility in the hips and ankles. Practice this pose regularly, focusing on stability and alignment, to cultivate strength, balance, and grace in your yoga practice.

Dolphin Pose (Ardha Pincha Mayurasana)

Dolphin Pose, or Ardha Pincha Mayurasana in Sanskrit, is a variation of Downward-Facing Dog that strengthens the arms, shoulders, and core while also stretching the hamstrings and calves. Here's how to practice it:

1. Begin on your hands and knees in a tabletop position on the mat, with your wrists directly under your shoulders and your knees directly under your hips.
2. Lower onto your forearms, bringing your elbows directly under your shoulders, with your forearms parallel to each other and your palms pressing firmly into the mat.
3. Tuck your toes under and lift your hips toward the ceiling, coming into a downward-facing dog position on your forearms.
4. Keep your knees bent slightly and your heels lifted off the mat, allowing your hips to lift upward.
5. Press down firmly through your forearms and lift through your

shoulders, creating space between your shoulder blades.

6. Engage your core muscles to support your spine, and lengthen through your tailbone, reaching it toward the ceiling.
7. Keep your neck relaxed and your gaze directed toward your feet or between your forearms.
8. Press firmly into your palms and forearms to lift your hips higher and stretch through your hamstrings and calves.
9. Hold the pose for 15-30 seconds, breathing deeply and evenly.
10. To release, exhale as you gently lower your knees back down to the mat, coming back to a tabletop position.

Dolphin Pose strengthens the arms, shoulders, and core muscles, while also stretching the hamstrings and calves. It can help improve upper body strength, shoulder stability, and flexibility in the spine and lower body. Practice this pose regularly, focusing on alignment and engagement of the core and shoulder muscles, to cultivate strength, stability, and balance in your yoga practice.

Revolved Triangle Pose (Parivrtta Trikonasana)

Revolved Triangle Pose, or Parivrtta Trikonasana in Sanskrit, is a powerful standing twist that strengthens the legs, stretches the hamstrings and hips, and improves spinal mobility and balance. Here's how to practice it:

1. Begin standing at the top of your mat in Mountain Pose (Tadasana), with your feet hip-width apart and your arms by your sides.
2. Step your left foot back about 3-4 feet and turn it out slightly, so your left toes point toward the left side of your mat at about a 45-degree angle.
3. Square your hips toward the front of your mat, keeping your left hip in line with your right hip.
4. On an inhale, reach your arms out to the sides at shoulder height, palms facing down, and gaze over your right fingertips.
5. On an exhale, hinge forward at your hips and begin to lower your torso toward your right leg, keeping your spine long and your chest lifted.

6. Bring your right hand to the outside of your right shin, ankle, or the floor, whichever is accessible to you. You can also place a block on the outside of your right foot for support.

7. Reach your left arm up toward the ceiling, with your biceps alongside your left ear and your palm facing down. Your left shoulder should be stacked directly over your right shoulder.

8. Keep your chest and hips open toward the side of your mat, and your spine lengthened from your tailbone to the crown of your head.

9. Gaze up toward your left hand, if it's comfortable for your neck.

10. Engage your core muscles to support your spine, and press down firmly through the outer edge of your left foot and the inner edge of your right foot to maintain stability.

11. Hold the pose for 15-30 seconds, breathing deeply and evenly.

12. To release, exhale as you bring your left hand back down to the mat and lift your torso back up to a standing position.

13. Repeat the pose on the other side, stepping your right foot back and

twisting toward the left side of your mat.

Revolved Triangle Pose strengthens the legs, stretches the hamstrings and hips, and improves spinal mobility and balance. It also stimulates the abdominal organs and can help improve digestion and elimination. Practice this pose regularly, focusing on lengthening through the spine and opening through the chest, to cultivate strength, flexibility, and balance in your yoga practice.

Revolved Chair Pose (Parivrtta Utkatasana)

Revolved Chair Pose, or Parivrtta Utkatasana in Sanskrit, is a challenging standing twist that strengthens the legs, core, and back muscles while also improving balance and flexibility. Here's how to practice it:

1. Begin standing at the top of your mat in Mountain Pose (Tadasana), with your feet hip-width apart and your arms by your sides.
2. Bend your knees and lower your hips down into Chair Pose (Utkatasana), as if you were sitting back into an imaginary chair. Keep your knees together and your weight in your heels.
3. On an inhale, reach your arms up alongside your ears, with your palms facing each other, and engage your core muscles to lengthen through your spine.
4. On an exhale, twist your torso to the right, bringing your left elbow to the outside of your right thigh. Your hands should be in prayer position, with your palms pressing together firmly.

5. Keep your knees and thighs pressing together and your hips squared forward as much as possible.
6. Press down through your feet to lift your chest and lengthen through your spine, maintaining a straight line from your tailbone to the crown of your head.
7. Keep your gaze steady and your breath smooth and steady.
8. If you're comfortable, you can gaze up toward the ceiling, bringing your twist deeper.
9. Hold the pose for 15-30 seconds, breathing deeply and evenly.
10. To release, inhale as you return to center, lifting your torso back up to Chair Pose.
11. Repeat the twist on the other side, bringing your right elbow to the outside of your left thigh.

Revolved Chair Pose strengthens the legs, core, and back muscles, while also improving balance and flexibility. It stimulates the abdominal organs and can help improve digestion and elimination. Practice this pose regularly, focusing on maintaining stability and alignment in the legs and spine, to cultivate strength, flexibility, and balance in your yoga practice.

Happy Baby Pose (Ananda Balasana)

Happy Baby Pose, or Ananda Balasana in Sanskrit, is a relaxing yoga pose that gently stretches the hips, groin, and lower back while also calming the mind and relieving stress. Here's how to practice it:

1. Begin by lying on your back on the mat with your knees bent and your feet flat on the floor.
2. Exhale as you hug your knees into your chest, bringing them toward your armpits.
3. Reach your hands to grab the outside edges of your feet or your ankles, with your palms facing up.
4. Flex your feet, pressing your heels toward the ceiling, and gently pull your knees down toward the mat, opening your hips.
5. Keep your tailbone grounded on the mat and your lower back pressing into the floor.
6. Relax your shoulders and neck, allowing them to soften and release any tension.
7. Keep your gaze soft and your face relaxed, breathing deeply and evenly.

8. You can gently rock from side to side or forward and backward to massage your spine and hips.

9. Hold the pose for 30 seconds to 1 minute, breathing deeply and allowing yourself to surrender fully to relaxation.

10. To release, exhale as you slowly release your feet and hug your knees back into your chest.

11. Extend your legs long on the mat and take a few deep breaths, allowing your body to relax completely in Corpse Pose (Savasana).

Happy Baby Pose gently stretches the hips, groin, and lower back, while also calming the mind and relieving stress. It can help release tension in the hips and lower back, improve flexibility, and promote relaxation and restful sleep. Practice this pose regularly, especially at the end of your yoga practice or before bedtime, to cultivate a sense of ease and well-being in your body and mind.

Wide-Legged Forward Bend (Prasarita Padottanasana)

Wide-Legged Forward Bend, or Prasarita Padottanasana in Sanskrit, is a rejuvenating yoga pose that stretches the hamstrings, calves, and lower back while also calming the mind and relieving stress. Here's how to practice it:

1. Begin standing at the top of your mat with your feet about 3-4 feet apart, parallel to each other.
2. Engage your quadriceps muscles and lift your kneecaps to activate your legs.
3. On an exhale, hinge forward at your hips and begin to fold forward, keeping your spine long and your chest open.
4. Bring your hands to the floor directly underneath your shoulders, or you can hold onto your ankles or shins if that feels more accessible.
5. Keep your head and neck relaxed, allowing your spine to lengthen and your torso to release toward the floor.
6. Press down through the outer edges of your feet and lift through your inner arches to engage your leg muscles.

7. Allow your hips to stack directly over your heels, and your weight to distribute evenly between your feet.
8. If you're comfortable, you can walk your hands back between your feet, bringing your head closer to the mat.
9. Hold the pose for 30 seconds to 1 minute, breathing deeply and evenly.
10. To release, inhale as you slowly lift your torso back up to a standing position, engaging your core muscles to support your spine.

Wide-Legged Forward Bend stretches the hamstrings, calves, and lower back, while also calming the mind and relieving stress. It can help improve flexibility in the legs and spine, alleviate tension in the lower back, and promote relaxation and grounding. Practice this pose regularly, focusing on maintaining length in the spine and openness in the chest, to cultivate a sense of ease and well-being in your body and mind.

Side Plank Pose (Vasisthasana)

Side Plank Pose, or Vasisthasana in Sanskrit, is a challenging arm balance that strengthens the arms, shoulders, core, and legs while also improving balance and concentration. Here's how to practice it:

1. Begin in a plank position, with your wrists directly under your shoulders and your body in a straight line from your head to your heels.
2. Shift your weight onto your right hand and outer edge of your right foot, coming onto the outer edge of your right foot and stacking your left foot on top of your right foot.
3. Engage your core muscles to stabilize your body, and lift your left arm up toward the ceiling, stacking your left shoulder directly over your right shoulder.
4. Keep your body in a straight line from your head to your heels, and avoid letting your hips sink or lift too high.
5. Press down firmly through your right hand and the outer edge of your right foot to lift your hips and create space in your side body.

6. Keep your gaze steady and your breath smooth and steady.
7. If you're comfortable, you can gaze up toward your left hand, bringing your twist deeper.
8. Hold the pose for 15-30 seconds, breathing deeply and evenly.
9. To release, exhale as you gently lower your left hand back down to the mat and return to a plank position.
10. Repeat the pose on the other side, shifting your weight onto your left hand and outer edge of your left foot, and lifting your right arm up toward the ceiling.

Side Plank Pose strengthens the arms, shoulders, core, and legs, while also improving balance, concentration, and coordination. It can help improve upper body strength, shoulder stability, and core stability. Practice this pose regularly, focusing on alignment and engagement of the core and shoulder muscles, to cultivate strength, stability, and balance in your yoga practice.

Revolved Side Angle Pose (Parivrtta Parsvakonasana)

Revolved Side Angle Pose, or Parivrtta Parsvakonasana in Sanskrit, is a dynamic standing twist that stretches the hips, thighs, and spine while also strengthening the legs and core muscles. Here's how to practice it:

1. Begin in a standing position at the top of your mat, with your feet together and your arms by your sides in Mountain Pose (Tadasana).
2. Step your left foot back about 3-4 feet and turn it out slightly, so your left toes point toward the left side of your mat at about a 45-degree angle.
3. Bend your right knee, stacking it directly over your right ankle, and lower your hips toward the floor, coming into a lunge position.
4. Ensure your left leg is straight and strong, with your left heel pressing into the mat.
5. On an inhale, reach your arms out to the sides at shoulder height, palms facing down, and gaze over your right fingertips.
6. On an exhale, twist your torso to the right, bringing your left elbow to the

outside of your right thigh. Your hands should be in prayer position, with your palms pressing together firmly.

7. Keep your knees and thighs pressing together and your hips squared forward as much as possible.

8. Press down through your feet to lift your chest and lengthen through your spine, maintaining a straight line from your tailbone to the crown of your head.

9. Keep your gaze steady and your breath smooth and steady.

10. If you're comfortable, you can gaze up toward the ceiling, bringing your twist deeper.

11. Hold the pose for 15-30 seconds, breathing deeply and evenly.

12. To release, inhale as you return to center, lifting your torso back up and bringing your hands to prayer position.

13. Repeat the twist on the other side, stepping your right foot back and twisting toward the left side of your mat.

Revolved Side Angle Pose stretches the hips, thighs, and spine, while also strengthening the legs and core muscles. It stimulates the abdominal organs and can help improve digestion and elimination. Practice this pose regularly, focusing on maintaining stability and alignment in the legs and spine, to cultivate strength, flexibility, and balance in your yoga practice.

Camel Pose (Ustrasana)

Camel Pose, or Ustrasana in Sanskrit, is a heart-opening backbend that stretches the front of the body, including the chest, abdomen, and hip flexors, while also strengthening the back muscles and improving spinal flexibility. Here's how to practice it:

1. Begin by kneeling on the mat with your knees hip-width apart and your thighs perpendicular to the floor. Ensure that your shins and feet are relaxed on the mat, with the tops of your feet pressing into the ground.
2. Place your hands on your lower back, fingers pointing downward, and thumbs resting on your sacrum. Your fingertips should be pointing toward your tailbone.
3. Engage your core muscles and gently press your hips forward, tilting your pelvis slightly forward.
4. On an inhale, lift your chest toward the ceiling, arching your back and bringing your shoulder blades together.
5. As you continue to lift your chest, reach your hands down toward your

heels, one at a time. If you can't reach your heels comfortably, keep your hands on your lower back for support.

6. Once your hands are on your heels, press your hips forward and lift your chest toward the ceiling, creating a deep arch in your upper back.
7. Keep your neck long and your head in a neutral position, avoiding any compression in the back of your neck.
8. If it's comfortable for your neck, you can drop your head back and gaze toward the wall behind you.
9. Hold the pose for 15-30 seconds, breathing deeply and evenly.
10. To release, exhale as you slowly bring your hands back to your lower back, one at a time, and lift your torso back up to a kneeling position.
11. Rest in Child's Pose (Balasana) for a few breaths to counterpose the backbend.

Camel Pose stretches the front of the body, including the chest, abdomen, and hip flexors, while also strengthening the back muscles and improving spinal flexibility. It opens the heart center, promotes emotional release, and stimulates the organs in the abdomen. Practice this pose mindfully, listening to your body and only going as deep into the pose as feels comfortable for you.

Cow Face Pose
(Gomukhasana)

Cow Face Pose, or Gomukhasana in Sanskrit, is a seated yoga pose that stretches the hips, thighs, chest, shoulders, and arms. It's named for the shape the legs and arms make, resembling the face of a cow. Here's how to practice it:

1. Begin seated on the mat with your legs extended in front of you.
2. Bend your knees and place your feet on the floor, hip-width apart.
3. Slide your left foot under your right knee and bring it to the outside of your right hip.
4. Cross your right leg over your left thigh, stacking your right knee directly on top of your left knee. Your right foot should be on the outside of your left hip.
5. Adjust your position so your sit bones are grounded evenly on the mat.
6. Inhale as you reach your left arm up toward the ceiling, then bend your left elbow and reach your hand down between your shoulder blades.

7. Inhale again as you reach your right arm out to the side at shoulder height, palm facing down.
8. Exhale and bend your right elbow, reaching your hand behind your back and clasping your fingers with your left hand. If you can't reach your fingers, you can use a strap or towel to hold onto.
9. Keep your spine long and your chest lifted as you gently press your elbows away from each other, feeling a stretch across your chest and shoulders.
10. Hold the pose for 15-30 seconds, breathing deeply and evenly.
11. To release, exhale as you gently release your hands and uncross your legs.
12. Repeat the pose on the other side, crossing your right foot under your left knee and stacking your left knee on top of your right knee.

Cow Face Pose stretches the hips, thighs, chest, shoulders, and arms, while also improving posture and increasing flexibility. It can help alleviate tension and discomfort in the hips and shoulders, and it's also beneficial for opening the chest and improving respiratory function. Practice this pose regularly, being mindful of any discomfort and using props or modifications as needed to support your practice.

Gate Pose (Parighasana)

Gate Pose, or Parighasana in Sanskrit, is a lateral stretch that stretches the sides of the body, opens the chest, and strengthens the legs. Here's how to practice it:

1. Begin by kneeling on the mat with your knees hip-width apart and your thighs perpendicular to the floor. Ensure that your shins and feet are relaxed on the mat, with the tops of your feet pressing into the ground.
2. Extend your right leg out to the side, with your foot flat on the mat and your toes pointing forward.
3. Press down through your right foot and engage your thigh muscles to stabilize your leg.
4. On an inhale, raise your arms out to the sides at shoulder height, palms facing down.
5. Exhale and reach your right hand down your right leg, sliding it down as far as comfortable. You can rest your hand on your shin, ankle, or the floor, whichever is accessible to you.
6. Extend your left arm overhead, reaching toward the right side, with your palm facing down.

7. Keep both arms in line with your shoulders, and avoid collapsing your chest forward.
8. Keep your gaze straight ahead or turn it upward toward your left hand.
9. Hold the pose for 15-30 seconds, breathing deeply and evenly.
10. To release, inhale as you slowly lift your torso back up to an upright position and bring your arms back to shoulder height.
11. Repeat the pose on the other side, extending your left leg out to the side and reaching your left hand down your left leg while extending your right arm overhead.

Gate Pose stretches the sides of the body, opens the chest, and strengthens the legs. It can help improve spinal flexibility, alleviate tension in the shoulders and chest, and increase overall mobility. Practice this pose mindfully, listening to your body and only going as far into the stretch as feels comfortable for you.

Dolphin Plank Pose (Makara Adho Mukha Svanasana)

Dolphin Plank Pose, also known as Makara Adho Mukha Svanasana in Sanskrit, is a variation of the traditional Plank Pose that strengthens the arms, shoulders, core, and legs. Here's how to practice it:

1. Begin by coming into a forearm plank position on the mat. Lower onto your forearms with your elbows directly under your shoulders and your hands clasped together or parallel to each other.
2. Extend your legs behind you, keeping them hip-width apart, and come onto the balls of your feet. Your body should form a straight line from your head to your heels.
3. Engage your core muscles to stabilize your spine and pelvis, and draw your shoulder blades down and back to open your chest.
4. Press down firmly through your forearms and lift your hips toward the ceiling, coming into a Dolphin Pose position. Your body should resemble an inverted "V" shape.

5. Keep your neck in line with your spine and your gaze directed between your forearms or toward your feet.
6. Press down through your heels to engage your leg muscles and lift your sitting bones toward the ceiling.
7. Hold the pose for 15-30 seconds, breathing deeply and evenly.
8. To release, exhale as you slowly lower your hips back down to the mat, coming back into a forearm plank position.
9. You can repeat the pose for additional rounds or move into a different posture.

Dolphin Plank Pose strengthens the arms, shoulders, core, and legs, while also improving balance and stability. It helps build endurance and stamina, tones the abdominal muscles, and improves posture. Practice this pose regularly, focusing on maintaining proper alignment and engaging the core and leg muscles, to cultivate strength and stability in your yoga practice.

Supported Shoulder Stand (Salamba Sarvangasana)

Supported Shoulder Stand, or Salamba Sarvangasana in Sanskrit, is an inverted yoga pose that provides numerous benefits, including improved circulation, relaxation, and relief from stress and fatigue. Here's how to practice it using props for support:

1. Begin by lying on your back on the mat with your knees bent and your feet flat on the floor.
2. Place a folded blanket or yoga bolster under your hips to provide support.
3. Gently lift your legs off the floor and bring your knees toward your chest.
4. Press your hands into the mat and lift your hips, allowing your legs to come overhead until your toes touch the floor behind you.
5. Use your hands to support your lower back and hips as you walk your hands up your back toward your shoulder blades.
6. Once your hands are in place, engage your core muscles and extend your legs upward toward the ceiling.

7. Keep your neck long and your gaze directed toward your chest or the ceiling.
8. Adjust the height of the support under your hips as needed to ensure your neck and spine are in a straight line.
9. Hold the pose for 30 seconds to 1 minute, breathing deeply and evenly.
10. To release, gently bend your knees and lower your feet back down toward the floor, one at a time.
11. Lower your hips back down onto the support, and then slowly roll onto your back.

Supported Shoulder Stand increases blood flow to the brain and thyroid gland, improves digestion, and relieves symptoms of stress, anxiety, and mild depression. It also stretches the shoulders and neck and strengthens the core muscles. Practice this pose mindfully, using props for support as needed, and avoid it if you have neck or spine injuries. Always listen to your body and work within your own limits.

Standing Forward Bend
(Uttanasana)

Standing Forward Bend, or Uttanasana in Sanskrit, is a rejuvenating yoga pose that stretches the entire back side of the body, including the spine, hamstrings, and calves. Here's how to practice it:

1. Begin standing tall at the top of your mat in Mountain Pose (Tadasana), with your feet hip-width apart and your arms by your sides.
2. Take a deep inhale to lengthen through your spine, lifting your chest and rolling your shoulders back.
3. Exhale and hinge forward at your hips, folding your torso over your legs.
4. Allow your knees to bend slightly if needed to maintain a straight spine.
5. Bring your hands to the floor beside your feet, or you can hold onto opposite elbows and gently sway from side to side to release tension in the spine.
6. Let your head hang heavy, releasing any tension in your neck and allowing your spine to lengthen.

7. Engage your quadriceps to gently lift your kneecaps and lengthen through the backs of your legs.

8. If it's comfortable for you, you can straighten your legs fully and bring your forehead toward your shins.

9. Relax your shoulders away from your ears and let your breath flow smoothly and deeply.

10. Hold the pose for 30 seconds to 1 minute, breathing deeply and allowing your body to soften and release with each exhale.

11. To release the pose, inhale as you slowly roll your spine up to a standing position, stacking each vertebra one at a time.

12. Take a moment to pause in Mountain Pose and notice the effects of the forward bend on your body and breath.

Standing Forward Bend stretches the entire back side of the body, including the spine, hamstrings, and calves. It also calms the mind and relieves stress and anxiety. Practice this pose regularly, focusing on maintaining a straight spine and deepening your breath, to cultivate flexibility and relaxation in your body and mind.

Reclining Hand-to-Big-Toe Pose (Supta Padangusthasana)

Reclining Hand-to-Big-Toe Pose, or Supta Padangusthasana in Sanskrit, is a gentle yoga pose that stretches the hamstrings, calves, and hips while also improving flexibility and relieving tension in the legs and lower back. Here's how to practice it:

1. Begin by lying on your back on the mat with your legs extended and your arms by your sides.
2. Bend your right knee and hug it into your chest, keeping your left leg extended on the mat.
3. Hold onto the big toe of your right foot with your right hand. If you can't reach your big toe, you can hold onto your ankle or calf instead.
4. Keep your left leg active and engaged, pressing your left heel firmly into the mat.
5. Straighten your right leg upward toward the ceiling, keeping it as straight as possible. If your leg doesn't straighten fully, you can keep a slight bend in the knee.

6. Flex your right foot and press through your heel, reaching it toward the ceiling.
7. Keep your left leg grounded and your hips level on the mat.
8. If it's comfortable for your neck, you can gently lift your head and shoulders off the mat, bringing your chin toward your chest.
9. Hold the pose for 30 seconds to 1 minute, breathing deeply and evenly.
10. To release, exhale as you gently release your right leg back down to the mat and hug both knees into your chest.
11. Repeat the pose on the other side, bending your left knee and extending your left leg upward toward the ceiling.

Reclining Hand-to-Big-Toe Pose stretches the hamstrings, calves, and hips, while also relieving tension in the legs and lower back. It can help improve flexibility and mobility in the legs and hips and promote relaxation and stress relief. Practice this pose regularly, focusing on deepening your breath and maintaining a sense of ease and relaxation in your body and mind.

Revolved Head-to-Knee Pose (Parivrtta Janu Sirsasana)

Revolved Head-to-Knee Pose, or Parivrtta Janu Sirsasana in Sanskrit, is a seated twist that stretches the spine, hamstrings, and hips while also improving digestion and detoxification. Here's how to practice it:

1. Begin seated on the mat with your legs extended in front of you and your spine tall.
2. Bend your right knee and bring the sole of your right foot to the inner left thigh, allowing your right knee to fall open to the side.
3. Ensure that your left leg remains extended and active on the mat, with your toes pointing up toward the ceiling.
4. On an inhale, reach your arms overhead, lengthening through your spine.
5. On an exhale, twist your torso to the left, bringing your left hand to the outside of your right knee and your right hand to the mat behind you.
6. Keep your left leg active and your left foot flexed.

7. Inhale to lengthen through your spine, and exhale to deepen the twist, gently pressing your right hand into the mat to help rotate your torso.
8. If it's comfortable for your neck, you can gaze over your left shoulder, deepening the twist.
9. Hold the pose for 30 seconds to 1 minute, breathing deeply and evenly.
10. To release, inhale as you slowly unwind the twist, coming back to center with your spine tall.
11. Repeat the pose on the other side, bending your left knee and twisting to the right.

Revolved Head-to-Knee Pose stretches the spine, hamstrings, and hips, while also stimulating the abdominal organs and improving digestion. It can help relieve tension in the back and hips and promote detoxification and cleansing in the body. Practice this pose mindfully, focusing on maintaining length in the spine and openness in the chest, to cultivate balance and harmony in your body and mind.

Standing Split Pose (Urdhva Prasarita Eka Padasana)

Standing Split Pose, or Urdhva Prasarita Eka Padasana in Sanskrit, is a balancing posture that stretches the hamstrings, calves, and hips while also improving balance and concentration. Here's how to practice it:

1. Begin standing tall at the top of your mat in Mountain Pose (Tadasana), with your feet hip-width apart and your arms by your sides.
2. Shift your weight onto your left foot and lift your right foot off the mat, bringing your right knee toward your chest.
3. On an exhale, begin to hinge forward at your hips, extending your right leg straight back behind you.
4. Keep your hips level and square to the front of your mat, with your right toes pointing toward the floor.
5. Engage your core muscles to stabilize your spine, and keep your chest lifted as you continue to fold forward.
6. Bring your hands to the mat or blocks on either side of your left foot for support.

7. Press down firmly through your hands and left foot to lift your right leg higher toward the ceiling.
8. Keep your left leg strong and engaged, pressing firmly into the mat.
9. Flex your right foot and reach through your right heel to lengthen your leg.
10. Keep your gaze steady and your breath smooth and steady.
11. Hold the pose for 15-30 seconds, breathing deeply and evenly.
12. To release, exhale as you gently lower your right foot back down to meet your left foot at the top of your mat.
13. Repeat the pose on the other side, shifting your weight onto your right foot and lifting your left leg up behind you.

Standing Split Pose stretches the hamstrings, calves, and hips, while also improving balance, concentration, and stability. It helps build strength and flexibility in the legs and core muscles and promotes a sense of grounding and presence. Practice this pose regularly, focusing on maintaining alignment and stability in the standing leg, to cultivate balance and awareness in your yoga practice.

Revolved Half Moon Pose (Parivrtta Ardha Chandrasana)

Revolved Half Moon Pose, or Parivrtta Ardha Chandrasana in Sanskrit, is a challenging standing balance pose that combines elements of balance, strength, and flexibility. Here's how to practice it:

1. Begin in a standing position at the top of your mat, with your feet together and your arms by your sides.
2. Shift your weight onto your right foot and begin to lift your left leg off the mat, coming into Half Moon Pose (Ardha Chandrasana). Keep your left leg lifted parallel to the floor and flex your left foot.
3. Place your left hand on the mat about a foot in front of your right foot, positioning it slightly to the left of your right foot.
4. Keep your right hand on your right hip to start.
5. On an exhale, begin to twist your torso to the right, opening your chest toward the right side of your mat.

6. As you twist, extend your right arm toward the ceiling, reaching it up and overhead.
7. Keep your left leg strong and engaged, pressing actively through the heel.
8. Engage your core muscles to maintain stability and balance.
9. Keep your gaze steady and your breath smooth and steady.
10. If it's comfortable for your neck, you can gaze up toward your right hand.
11. Hold the pose for 15-30 seconds, breathing deeply and evenly.
12. To release, exhale as you slowly lower your right hand back down to the mat and return to Half Moon Pose.
13. Lower your left leg back down to the mat and come back to standing at the top of your mat.
14. Repeat the pose on the other side, shifting your weight onto your left foot and lifting your right leg.

Revolved Half Moon Pose strengthens the legs, core, and stabilizing muscles, while also improving balance, concentration, and spinal mobility. It stretches the hips, hamstrings, and side body, and it can help improve digestion and detoxification. Practice this pose mindfully, focusing on maintaining stability and alignment, to cultivate strength, flexibility, and balance in your yoga practice.

Camel Pose (Ustrasana)

Camel Pose, or Ustrasana in Sanskrit, is a powerful backbend that stretches the front of the body while also opening the chest, shoulders, and throat. Here's how to practice it:

1. Begin by kneeling on the mat with your knees hip-width apart. Ensure your thighs are perpendicular to the floor, and your shins and the tops of your feet are resting on the mat.
2. Place your hands on your lower back, fingers pointing downward, and thumbs resting on your sacrum. Your fingertips should be pointing toward your tailbone.
3. On an inhale, engage your core muscles and slowly start to arch backward, pressing your hips forward.
4. As you continue to lean back, reach your hands down one at a time to grasp your heels. If you can't reach your heels, keep your hands on your lower back for support.
5. Once your hands are on your heels, press your hips forward and lift your chest toward the ceiling, allowing

your head to drop back if it feels comfortable for your neck.

6. Keep your thighs perpendicular to the floor and your shoulder blades drawn together to open your chest.
7. If it feels comfortable, you can allow your head to drop back and gaze behind you, keeping your neck relaxed.
8. Hold the pose for 15-30 seconds, breathing deeply and evenly.
9. To release, exhale as you slowly bring your hands back to your lower back one at a time, and then lift your torso back up to an upright position.
10. Sit back on your heels and take a moment to rest in Child's Pose (Balasana), allowing your spine to neutralize.

Camel Pose stretches the front of the body, including the chest, abdomen, and hip flexors, while also strengthening the back muscles and improving spinal flexibility. It can help improve posture, alleviate back pain, and stimulate the abdominal organs. Practice this pose mindfully, focusing on lengthening through the spine and opening through the chest, to cultivate strength, flexibility, and balance in your yoga practice.

Fire Log Pose
(Agnistambhasana)

Fire Log Pose, or Agnistambhasana in Sanskrit, is a seated yoga pose that stretches the hips, groins, and glutes. It is also known as Double Pigeon Pose. Here's how to practice it:

1. Begin seated on the mat with your legs extended in front of you.
2. Bend your right knee and bring your right foot to the outside of your left hip, with your right shin parallel to the front edge of the mat.
3. Stack your left shin on top of your right shin, bringing your left ankle to the outside of your right knee. Your left knee should be directly above your right ankle.
4. Flex both feet to protect your knees.
5. If your hips are tight, you may need to adjust the position of your feet to find a comfortable position.
6. Sit up tall with a straight spine, and place your hands on your knees or on the mat beside your hips for support.
7. If you're comfortable, you can hinge forward at the hips, folding your torso over your legs.

8. Keep your spine long and your chest lifted as you fold forward.
9. Hold the pose for 30 seconds to 1 minute, breathing deeply and evenly.
10. To release, inhale as you slowly lift your torso back up to an upright position.
11. Unwind your legs and extend them out in front of you.
12. Repeat the pose on the other side, bending your left knee and stacking your left shin on top of your right shin.

Fire Log Pose stretches the hips, groins, and glutes, while also improving flexibility and mobility in the hip joints. It can help alleviate tension and discomfort in the hips and lower back, and it's also beneficial for improving posture and increasing circulation in the lower body. Practice this pose regularly, focusing on maintaining length in the spine and openness in the hips, to cultivate ease and comfort in your body and mind.

One-Legged King Pigeon Pose (Eka Pada Rajakapotasana)

One-Legged King Pigeon Pose, or Eka Pada Rajakapotasana in Sanskrit, is an intermediate to advanced yoga pose that deeply stretches the hips, thighs, groins, abdomen, chest, shoulders, and neck. Here's how to practice it:

1. Begin in a tabletop position on the mat, with your wrists directly under your shoulders and your knees directly under your hips.
2. Slide your right knee forward toward your right wrist and angle your right shin under your torso, bringing your right foot toward your left hip. Your right knee should be positioned toward the outer edge of the mat.
3. Extend your left leg straight back behind you, lowering your hips toward the mat. Ensure your left hip is squared toward the front of the mat.
4. Flex your left foot to protect your knee and engage your left quadriceps.
5. Inhale as you lift your chest and lengthen your spine.

6. On an exhale, begin to walk your hands forward, folding forward over your right shin.

7. Rest your forearms on the mat and relax your forehead toward the ground. If you're able to go deeper, you can extend your arms fully and bring your forehead to the mat.

8. Keep your hips level and square to the front of the mat, avoiding any twisting or rotation.

9. Hold the pose for 30 seconds to 1 minute, breathing deeply and evenly.

10. To release, inhale as you slowly walk your hands back toward your body, lifting your torso upright.

11. Return to tabletop position and repeat the pose on the other side, bringing your left knee forward and extending your right leg back.

One-Legged King Pigeon Pose deeply stretches the hips, thighs, groins, abdomen, chest, shoulders, and neck. It stimulates the abdominal organs and can help alleviate tension and discomfort in the hips and lower back. This pose also opens the heart and promotes emotional release. Practice it mindfully, listening to your body and honoring its limits, to cultivate balance, flexibility, and peace in your yoga practice.

Wide-Angle Seated Forward Bend (Upavistha Konasana)

Wide-Angle Seated Forward Bend, or Upavistha Konasana in Sanskrit, is a seated yoga pose that stretches the hamstrings, inner thighs, and groins while also opening the hips and lengthening the spine. Here's how to practice it:

1. Begin seated on the mat with your legs extended wide apart, as wide as comfortable for you. Flex your feet, with your toes pointing up toward the ceiling.
2. Sit up tall with a straight spine, and engage your quadriceps to help lift your kneecaps and lengthen through the backs of your legs.
3. Place your hands on the mat beside your hips for support.
4. On an inhale, lengthen through your spine, lifting your chest toward the ceiling.
5. On an exhale, begin to hinge forward at your hips, leading with your chest.
6. Keep your spine long as you fold forward, walking your hands forward on the mat.

7. Keep your toes pointing up toward the ceiling and your feet flexed to protect your knees.

8. You can rest your hands on the mat in front of you, or you can hold onto your shins, ankles, or feet, depending on your flexibility.

9. Allow your head to relax and your neck to release as you fold forward.

10. Keep your breath smooth and steady as you hold the pose.

11. Hold the pose for 30 seconds to 1 minute, breathing deeply and evenly.

12. To release, inhale as you slowly walk your hands back toward your body, lifting your torso back up to an upright position.

13. Bring your legs together and give them a gentle shake to release any tension.

Wide-Angle Seated Forward Bend stretches the hamstrings, inner thighs, and groins, while also opening the hips and lengthening the spine. It can help improve flexibility in the legs and hips and relieve tension in the lower back. Practice this pose regularly, focusing on maintaining length in the spine and openness in the hips, to cultivate ease and comfort in your body and mind.

One-Legged Forward Bend
(Janu Sirsasana)

One-Legged Forward Bend, or Janu Sirsasana in Sanskrit, is a seated yoga pose that stretches the hamstrings, calves, and spine while also providing a gentle massage to the abdominal organs. Here's how to practice it:

1. Begin seated on the mat with your legs extended in front of you.
2. Bend your right knee and bring the sole of your right foot to the inner left thigh. Allow your right knee to fall open to the side, so the sole of your right foot rests against your left inner thigh.
3. Ensure that your left leg remains extended and active on the mat, with your toes pointing up toward the ceiling.
4. Sit up tall with a straight spine, and engage your quadriceps to help lift your kneecaps and lengthen through the backs of your legs.
5. On an inhale, raise your arms overhead, lengthening through your spine.

6. On an exhale, begin to hinge forward at your hips, leading with your chest.
7. Keep your spine long as you fold forward, walking your hands forward on the mat.
8. Keep your toes pointing up toward the ceiling and your left foot flexed to protect your knee.
9. You can rest your hands on the mat in front of you, or you can hold onto your left shin, ankle, or foot, depending on your flexibility.
10. Allow your head to relax and your neck to release as you fold forward.
11. Keep your breath smooth and steady as you hold the pose.
12. Hold the pose for 30 seconds to 1 minute, breathing deeply and evenly.
13. To release, inhale as you slowly walk your hands back toward your body, lifting your torso back up to an upright position.
14. Extend your right leg back out in front of you and give it a gentle shake to release any tension.
15. Repeat the pose on the other side, bending your left knee and folding forward over your left leg.

One-Legged Forward Bend stretches the hamstrings, calves, and spine, while also providing a gentle massage to the abdominal organs. It can help improve flexibility in the legs and spine and relieve tension in the lower back. Practice this pose regularly, focusing on maintaining length in the spine and openness in the hips, to cultivate ease and comfort in your body and mind.

Shoulder Stand
(Sarvangasana)

Shoulder Stand, or Sarvangasana in Sanskrit, is an inverted yoga pose that offers a multitude of benefits, including improved circulation, thyroid function, and overall relaxation. Here's how to practice it safely:

1. Begin by lying flat on your back on your mat with your arms beside your body, palms facing down.
2. On an inhale, engage your core muscles and gently lift your legs off the mat, bringing them toward the ceiling.
3. Use your hands to support your lower back as you lift your hips off the mat, bringing your torso and legs into a vertical position.
4. Keep your elbows shoulder-width apart on the mat and your hands supporting your lower back.
5. Press your arms and hands firmly into the mat to lift your torso and legs higher, coming into a straight line from your shoulders to your heels.
6. Keep your neck long and your gaze directed toward your chest or the ceiling.

7. Engage your leg muscles to keep your legs active and your feet flexed.
8. Hold the pose for 30 seconds to 1 minute, breathing deeply and evenly.
9. To release, exhale as you slowly lower your legs back down to the mat, one at a time, and then lower your hips back down.
10. Lie flat on your back for a few breaths, allowing your body to rest and relax.

Shoulder Stand increases blood flow to the brain and thyroid gland, improves digestion, and relieves symptoms of stress and fatigue. It also stretches the shoulders and neck and strengthens the core and legs. Practice this pose mindfully, paying attention to your body's alignment and any sensations you experience, and avoid it if you have neck or spine injuries. Always listen to your body and work within your own limits.

Book description.

"Embark on a transformative journey to wellness with 'The Ultimate Guide to Yoga Poses.' This comprehensive book offers an immersive exploration of 50 yoga poses, each accompanied by detailed step-by-step instructions and vivid illustrations. Whether you're a beginner or an experienced practitioner, you'll find something to enhance your practice. From rejuvenating standing poses like Mountain and Warrior, to calming seated stretches like Lotus and Forward Bend, each pose is carefully explained to help you achieve optimal alignment and mindfulness. With this indispensable guide, you'll unlock the full potential of your yoga practice and cultivate a deeper connection between mind, body, and spirit."

www.ingramcontent.com/pod-product-compliance
Lightning Source LLC
Chambersburg PA
CBHW071039250726
48653CB00005B/1907